The Feel Well Project

*Experiments in Learning How
to Eat, Live and Think*

Lily Milkovic, NTP
and
Jenny Swain, NTP

BALBOA.
PRESS

A DIVISION OF HAY HOUSE

Balboa Press books may be ordered through
booksellers or by contacting:

Balboa Press
A Division of Hay House
1663 Liberty Drive
Bloomington, IN 47403
www.balboapress.com
1 (877) 407-4847

Because of the dynamic nature of the Internet, any web
addresses or links contained in this book may have changed
since publication and may no longer be valid. The views
expressed in this work are solely those of the author and do
not necessarily reflect the views of the publisher, and the
publisher hereby disclaims any responsibility for them.

The author of this book does not dispense medical advice or prescribe
the use of any technique as a form of treatment for physical, emotional,
or medical problems without the advice of a physician, either directly
or indirectly. The intent of the author is only to offer information
of a general nature to help you in your quest for emotional and
spiritual well-being. In the event you use any of the information
in this book for yourself, which is your constitutional right, the
author and the publisher assume no responsibility for your actions.

Any people depicted in stock imagery provided by Thinkstock are
models, and such images are being used for illustrative purposes only.
Certain stock imagery © Thinkstock.

Print information available on the last page.

ISBN: 978-1-5043-5742-5 (sc)
ISBN: 978-1-5043-5743-2 (e)

Balboa Press rev. date: 07/11/2016

Contents

Introduction

When I began my journey to recovery from an autoimmune disease I sought the direction of my naturopathic doctor, the advice of various books, blogs, articles and audio recordings and hung desperately on the words and wisdom of my favorite spiritual teachers. I felt like a sponge, desperate to soak up the answers from *someone*. *Anyone* that knew more. *Anyone* that appeared confident. *Anyone* that could promise a clear path to wellness.

At times I was conflicted. While my doctor told me I could eat all the grains my heart desired, for example, my research yielded different results. *Everyone* had an opinion. An opinion backed by sound reason and research. It was tough to find clear-cut answers to my questions, and it wasn't until I started experimenting that I found answers. I paid attention to how small changes affected me and discovered that the answers were inside *me* all along.

My drive to heal eventually led me to study nutritional therapy where I met fellow health-enthusiast and co-author of this book, Jenny Swain. Jenny's journey began after watching her father lose his battle with pancreatic cancer *and* experiencing a cancer scare of her own. Jenny began a quest to change her family history using the power of nutrition. By experimenting with different ways of eating and managing stress, Jenny determined what did and did not work to attain optimal health.

As Nutritional Therapists, Jenny and I prescribe to bio-individuality—the idea that each of us has a unique set of dietary and lifestyle needs based on metabolism and ancestry. There is no one-size-fits-all diet. Two people can eat the same diet with different outcomes. For this reason, it is important that we are able to discern what is best for ourselves without solely relying on external resources. *But, how do we do that?!*

To answer this question, we developed *The Feel Well Project.*

Imagine experimenting with making just one change to your diet or lifestyle while paying close attention to how it affects you. What could you learn about yourself? This is the essence of *The Feel Well Project*—52 simple, yet empowering, experiments in diet and lifestyle that teach you to tune in to your body's subtle cues. Gain the ability to make better choices for your health with *The Feel Well Project.*

We invite you to experiment with how different ways of eating, living and thinking affect you physically, mentally and spiritually.

Feel Well!

How to Use The Feel Well Project

The experiments in this book are organized in a progressive, cumulative nature. You will spend one full week on each experiment. There are two ways to use this book.

(1) Go through the book week by week in sequential order starting with experiment #1.

or

(2) Flip the pages and choose an experiment that energetically suits your needs.

It is highly recommended to start with #1 and progress week by week in sequential order. You might choose to practice *only* the experiment of the week or combine previous experiments with the current week's experiment for an enriching experience. Use the space provided under each experiment to log your experiences and discoveries.

There is no wrong way to use the Feel Well Project. After all, this is your experience and you know best.

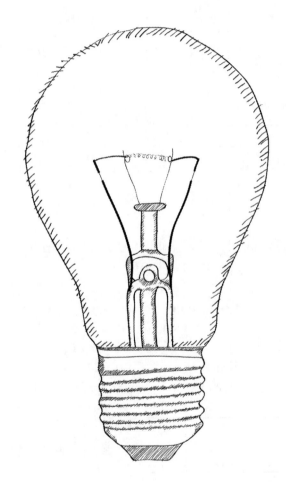

Experiment

noun
Pronunciation: /ikˈsper-ə-mənt/
A controlled procedure carried out to
discover, test, or demonstrate something.[1]

#1

Drink 20 Ounces of Water Every Morning

Water delivers oxygen to cells for energy, assists in detoxification, transports hormones and lubricates joints and tissues. It's the elixir of life!

After a night's rest, your body is dehydrated and needs water to jumpstart metabolism, get the bowels moving and energize itself for the day.

Experiment with drinking at least 20 oz. of pure, room temperature water upon rising and before any other food or drink. This addition to your morning ritual will start your day right.

What differences did you notice after drinking water every morning for a week?

#2

Breathe Deeply

Right now, without changing a thing, notice your breath.

Is it shallow or deep? Slow or fast? Does your belly expand as you inhale? Can you feel air move through your nasal passages?

Deliberate, deep breathing calms and centers the mind, relaxes the body, oxygenates blood, boosts the immune system and brings you into the present moment.

Experiment with this deep breathing exercise each day:

> Find a comfortable seated position, sit tall and root your feet to the ground. Close your eyes.
>
> Take a deep breath in through your nose for four counts, breathing deep into your belly, allowing it to expand fully, then breathing into your ribs allowing them to open and expand, and then into your chest.
>
> Exhale out your mouth for six counts, releasing the breath in the opposite direction—chest, ribs, and then belly.

Do this five or more times before opening your eyes. Remember: breathe in for four, breathe out for six.

How did this experiment make you feel?

#3

Eat Until You Are 80% Full

When you eat, your digestive enzymes do a happy dance. They get to work, breaking down your food into nutrients for bodily energy. However, eating until you're stuffed can leave you sluggish and uncomfortable. The enzymes can't do their job efficiently, and this leads to problems down the line.

After each bite this week, check in with your level of fullness. Stop eating when you feel about 80% full. This means that you're satiated but not stuffed. Put it this way—if you have to unbutton your pants after a meal... you probably ate too much! Be careful, sometimes the difference between satisfied at 80% and stuffed at 100% is only a bite or two.

What did you learn from this experiment?

#4

Take a Daily Walk Outside

The sounds of nature and the scent of fresh air are good for your soul. Nature connects you with a higher purpose and reminds you that the universe is awash with possibility.

Take 30 minutes each day to explore the outside world on a brisk walk. Notice your surroundings. Observe the crackle of leaves, birds flying overhead, the feel of a gentle breeze or the sound of your feet treading the ground.

Document your experience and observations here.

#5

Log Your Food

Keep a record this week of everything you put in your mouth. Whether it is food, drink, gum or candy, write it down and be honest! Additionally, note below how you feel after eating each meal or snack. Log your emotional and physical responses.

For example, after breakfast you might note that you experienced a stomach ache or fatigue, or perhaps you felt satiated and well-fueled to take on the day.

At the end of the week, review your log and draw conclusions. Can you connect headaches, heart palpitations, bloating or other digestive issues to certain foods? Which times of the day are easiest to make healthy choices? Do you skip breakfast? Do you eat three square meals or snack all day? Do you eat only when you are hungry or are there emotional reasons you turn to food? Are you satisfied with your choices? Is there room for improvement? Are there certain foods that make you feel good and others that don't?

#6

Eat Breakfast

It has been said that breakfast is the most important meal of the day, but all too often it is the most skipped meal of the day.

This week, eat breakfast every morning within one hour of rising. Do it *even* if you are not hungry.

Document how eating breakfast impacts your day. Notice how a protein-rich breakfast such as eggs or bacon makes you feel versus a carbohydrate-heavy breakfast of cereal or toast.

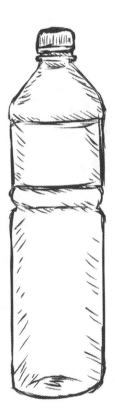

#7

Get Properly Hydrated

Water is all around us. Roughly 71% of the Earth's surface is water. We swim and bathe in it. We use it to cook. We nourish our plants and pets with it. No doubt, water plays an integral role in our lives. Why then, do we forget to drink enough of it?

Did you know that if you are even 2% dehydrated you will feel fatigued? Or that anxiety and headaches can result from simply not drinking enough water? A dehydrated body is susceptible to pain disorders, stress, depression, high blood pressure, hypertension, elevated blood cholesterol, excess body weight, edema, arthritis, asthma and allergies and even Alzheimer's!

Drink half your body weight in ounces of pure water each day (not to exceed 100 oz per day). For example, a 140 lb person should drink at least 70 oz of water per day (140/2=70).

Note: If you enjoy dehydrating beverages such as coffee, tea, alcohol and juice, you will need to increase your minimum requirement by about 24 oz.

TIP: You know you are well-hydrated when your urine is a pale yellow color.

Notice how seven days of proper hydration makes you feel.

#8

Write a Thank You Letter

Doesn't it feel amazing when people help you, compliment you or lift you up? Maybe they don't even realize what they did for you or how meaningful it was.

This week is your chance to let them know. Take time to write a heartfelt thank you letter, explaining how they lifted your spirits or made you feel important. There are probably multiple people in your life that have made you feel special – write them all if you wish!

Pausing to thank someone can be rewarding, or perhaps the experience might make you feel introspective or even vulnerable.

Document your experience below.

#9

Chew Your Food

Chew, chew, chew your food. How many times do you chew before swallowing? Is it at least 20 times? Most of us treat mealtime like a race, getting it done as fast as possible to move on to the next activity.

The simple act of chewing is one of the first steps in proper digestion. Your teeth break down large food molecules into smaller ones, while enzymes in your saliva lubricate the food, contributing to this breakdown. This aids the digestive process, making nutrients easier to absorb and assimilate.

During meals this week, put your fork down between bites and consciously chew 20 times before swallowing.

Document the experience here. Was this easy? Did you find it challenging? What digestive changes, if any, did you notice?

#10

Explore a Health Food Store

One way to learn about food labels, discover new products and find meal inspiration is to dedicate some time to it.

Spend 15 minutes perusing a health food store. This is not your weekly shopping trip. Arrive with the sole purpose to *EXPLORE*. Pick up products that interest you, read labels and allow your creative cooking juices to flow.

Take a few minutes to document your health food store exploration.

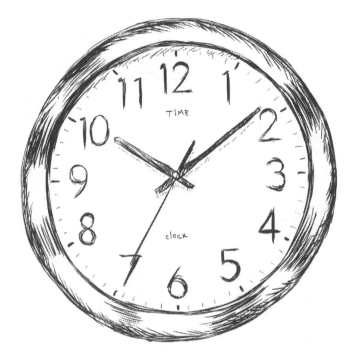

#11

Lights out by 10pm

You've heard the saying, "Early to bed, early to rise, makes a (wo)man healthy, wealthy and wise!" It is TRUE!

Hitting the hay consistently by 10pm supports your body's natural circadian rhythm. This optimizes hormone production, lowers risk of illness and leads to higher cognitive function, improved mood and enhanced energy levels.

This week, focus on being in bed with the lights out by 10pm. You may need to rework your schedule to make this possible, so be sure to plan accordingly.

Notice and document how this change at night affects your days.

#12

Eat Your Veggies

Unfortunately, vegetables have taken a backseat in our diets due to our culture's infatuation with fast and processed food. These plant foods, however, provide life-giving vitamins, minerals and fiber, allowing us to function at our best.

This week, challenge yourself to eat at *least* three different vegetables each day. Make your plate colorful with a rainbow of green, yellow and red, and it goes without saying that organic is always best.

To get started, here is a short list of vegetables to consider: carrots, broccoli, cauliflower, beets, kale, spinach, Brussels sprouts, cabbage, eggplant, tomatoes, okra, celery, turnips, zucchini, bell peppers, yellow squash, onions and garlic.

How did it go? What did you eat?

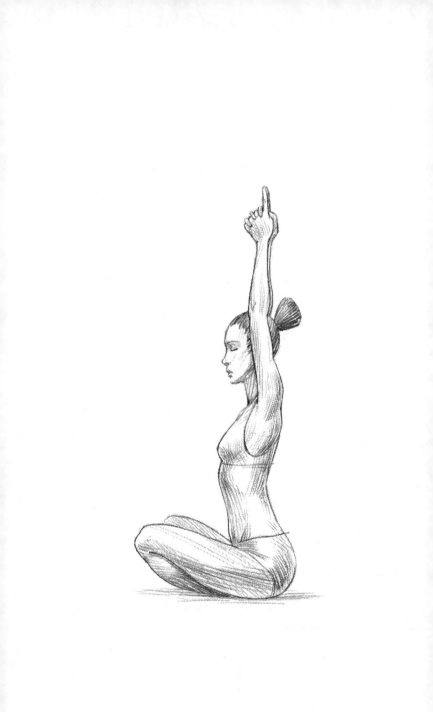

#13

Try a New Exercise Class

As they sing in the movie *Madagascar*, "I like to move it, move it," we should all enjoy moving our body. Exercise is important to overall health. In addition to the obvious benefit of improved physical condition, regular workouts promote organ detoxification, enhanced mood, restful sleep and increased energy. Your body needs to move, and you should have fun doing it.

Attend a different exercise class this week. Get out of your comfort zone. Need some ideas? Consider hiking, kickboxing, Pilates, spin, weight-training, water aerobics, a dance class or yoga. Better yet, grab a friend and have twice the fun!

The sky is the limit! Now, get moving! Record your exercise adventure below.

#14

Cut Out Alcohol

We know that alcohol isn't a health drink, but many of us choose to imbibe anyway. Alcohol dehydrates us, contributes to disturbed sleep patterns and burdens the liver—among many other things.

For one week, refrain from all alcohol. Skip the happy hour, cork up the wine and don't tap the beer keg.

If this experiment makes you anxious, ask yourself, "*Why?*" Instead of reaching for that drink, ponder why you need it in the first place. What body sensations, thoughts and emotions are you experiencing?

#15

Don't Take Things Personally

Sometimes people get under your skin, right? It is easy to get swept up and take things personally, but what if you told yourself that other people's words and actions have less to do with you and more to do with something *they're* dealing with?

This week, be immune to the actions and words of others. Notice when people or events get under your skin and acknowledge that it's probably not about you. Consciously choose to move on because it is truly not important what others think of you.

Take a few moments to write about your experiences.

#16

Don't Eat Past 5pm

Sleeping doesn't just refresh the mind and body. While you slumber, your body detoxifies and repairs itself. Going to bed with a full stomach leaves it focused on digesting rather than healing.

Avoid eating after 5:00pm every day this week. You may find you feel lighter, experience better bowl movements or sleep more soundly.

Log your experience here.

#17

Nix the Negative Self-Talk

You've let it happen. Maybe more than once. Maybe more than a thousand times. You've let that pesky inner voice spew its negativity, disrupt your self-confidence and leave you feeling small.

We often fail to realize the frequency and intensity in which we berate ourselves—both quietly in passing and out loud to others. Negative self-talk greatly impacts our self-worth and happiness.

This week, practice refraining from negative self-talk. Notice when it happens and make a concerted effort to stop.

Write your observations here.

#18

Be Silent

When you stop talking, you start listening.

Taking a vow of prolonged silence (both verbal and written communication) can be enlightening. A conscious choice to periodically refrain from communication with others shifts you into a more thoughtful mode. You can simply observe the world around you and acknowledge and process your inner feelings.

Schedule one or more days to practice silence. If this isn't possible, research and sign up for a future silent retreat.

Note your experience. What did you find most challenging? What emotions came to light? What did you learn from this experiment?

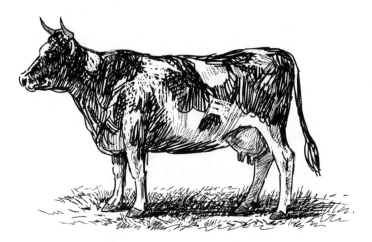

#19

Ditch the Dairy

Many people are sensitive to dairy. They don't realize that it is causing a stuffy nose, sore joints, uncomfortable digestion and bad skin.

Dairy's lactose and casein are the typical culprits. Lactose is problematic when a person doesn't produce the digestive enzyme lactase. Casein, a milk protein, causes trouble for people who are intolerant or sensitive to it.

Often we don't know how a food affects us until we remove it from our diet for a period of time.

For this week, avoid dairy and note whether or not you feel different.

Examples of dairy products include milk, cheese, butter, cream and yogurt. Be careful of foods with hidden dairy!

#20

Contemplate Humanity

Visit a busy place (i.e., a mall, an airport or a park on a nice day) just to observe other people. While watching, note how their lives must be different from yours and every stranger around them. If you desire, create imaginary lives for them while you observe.

The point of this experiment is to realize how different we are from each other and to generate empathy for others. We all have unique struggles, challenges, successes and victories. Be reminded of Plato's famous quote, "Be kind, for everyone you meet is fighting a hard battle."

Journal about your experience here.

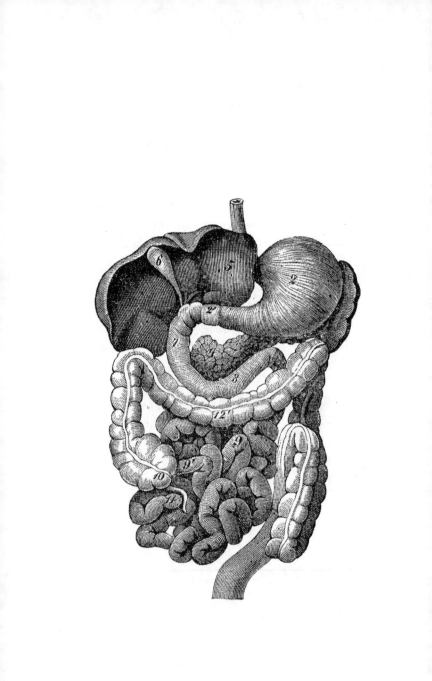

#21

Support Your Digestion

Proper digestion is a key foundation to good health. If you're not properly digesting, you're not reaping the benefits of the nutrients consumed.

How do you know if you need digestive support? Heartburn, belching, gas, bloating and stomach ache after eating are some indicators that support is needed. Common household products like lemon juice and apple cider vinegar are effective digestive aids.

Lemon contains citrus flavanols that stimulate the liver and support hydrochloric acid (HCl) production in the stomach. Despite what you may have heard, a substantial amount of HCl is needed for the proper breakdown of food. Apple cider vinegar also encourages HCl production and assists with protein breakdown.

This week, experiment with drinking at least one glass of water with the juice of an organic lemon each morning. Before every meal, mix a tablespoon or more of apple cider vinegar into a glass of water and sip 20 minutes before eating.

Take note of how you feel each day.

#22

Get in Alignment

Mahatma Gandhi once said, "Happiness is when what you think, what you say and what you do are in harmony."

Are the words you speak in alignment with your truth? Are you authentic in your actions?

For example, have you ever dreaded a social event that you agreed to attend, preferring to spend the night curled up on the couch with a good book? It is okay to politely decline invitations if they don't align with how you want to spend your time. Your time and energy is precious and nicely saying "no" to things creates time and space for what matters most.

Perhaps you find yourself being asked to lie and this goes against your moral code—can you be true to your values? Or perhaps someone undermines you—can you confront them in a non-contentious manner?

It is okay to be yourself. There is great peace and freedom that comes from being yourself—in thoughts, words and actions.

This week, notice areas in your life that don't align with your truth. Need some help? Start by writing down your truths. Truths are morals and values that make *you* who you are. Next, make a list of routine thoughts, words and actions that come up in your life. Spend time evaluating whether your responses support your internal beliefs.

#23

Cut Ties with TV and Social Media

You may spend more hours checking social media and watching TV than you realize or care to admit.

How does TV and social media make you feel...or *not* feel?

This week, if only for a day, cut ties with TV and social media outlets. Read, journal, nap, spend time with pets or have lunch with a friend instead.

Note what feelings and experiences come up.

#24

Eat Home-Cooked Meals

Commercially prepared foods are high in poor quality fats, sodium, sugar, additives and preservatives. Conversely, home-cooked meals are more nutritious because they contain fresher, less-processed ingredients. This gives you more control over what goes into your body.

Home-cooking also trains your palate to enjoy healthier fare by avoiding excitatory ingredients like MSG and sugar found in many restaurant meals.

This week, eat only home-cooked meals. You will find that a little planning can go a long way. Look up meal-planning or batch cooking recipes, pack your lunch and keep things simple—no need for elaborate four-course meals!

#25

Take an Epsom Salt Bath

Relax your nervous system, soothe your muscles and draw out toxins with a rewarding Epsom salt bath.

Add two cups of Epsom salt to a hot bath and soak for 20 minutes. If you don't have a tub, try a foot soak.

This week indulge in several Epsom salt baths.

Notice how you feel.

#26

Eat ONLY When You Are Hungry

Often we eat for reasons other than true hunger. We eat out of boredom, to self-soothe, to celebrate or to protect ourselves from feeling deeper emotions.

This week, challenge yourself to eat only when your stomach growls. If a piece of chicken and broccoli doesn't sound appetizing, you are not experiencing true hunger.

When you find yourself eating for reasons other than true hunger, consider WHY you eat. Keep a food journal noting what you ate and why. Some WHY examples might be fatigue, boredom, sadness, anxiety, happiness, celebration, social obligation, or procrastination. Instead of food, ask yourself what you hunger for. What do you really need? A hug? A nap? A talk with someone?

What did this experiment teach you?

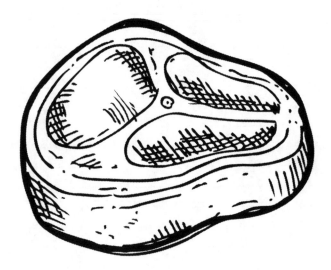

#27

Go Sans Meat

Animal products, especially red meat, have become a source of controversy. A Google search asking the question, "Is meat good for you," yields 278 million results with differing opinions.

Science indicates that meat provides beneficial amino acids required for the growth and repair of muscles, hormones, enzymes and antibodies, but how much meat do we really need?

Some cultures and schools of thought place an emphasis on high meat consumption, while others lean towards smaller quantities. For example, the Paleo community enjoys a high meat diet while vegetarians lean toward plant-based fare. Some people need more meat to feel sustained, while others need substantially less. Additionally, people with impaired digestion cannot assimilate larger portions of meat.

While eliminating meat once in a while works as a gentle detox, you may feel better eating it on a regular basis. The question then becomes, "how much?"

For this week, go without meat and notice how you feel.

#28

Don't Make Assumptions

An assumption is defined as "a thing that is accepted as true or as certain to happen, *without proof*" (emphasis mine). We tend to see and hear what we want. Without realizing, we make assumptions, draw conclusions and feel dissatisfied in our interactions with others.

These assumptions can be a source of pain and drama—especially if inaccurate. This week, be aware of the assumptions you find yourself making and notice how they make you feel. What would happen if, instead of assuming a particular meaning and blindly responding to that meaning, you asked for clarification?

This week, find the courage to ask questions instead of jumping to conclusions. Make a few journal entries about your experiences.

#29

Be a Do-Gooder

"The purpose of human life is to serve and to show compassion and the will to help others." – Albert Schweitzer

Find ways to help others this week. You can cook a meal for someone in need, run an elderly person's errands, help a non-profit organization with a project, volunteer at an animal shelter or perform any other activity that speaks to your heart.

What did you do and how did it make you feel?

#30

Avoid Using the Microwave Oven

Convenient? Yes. Safe? Questionable. Microwave ovens, developed in the 1950s, have been shown to destroy nutrients in food. According to the *Journal of the Science of Food and Agriculture*, broccoli cooked by microwave loses up to 97 percent of its antioxidants. Microwaves work by channeling heat energy directly into the molecules inside food. They do this much like the sun heats your face – by radiation. Microwave ovens are surrounded by strong metal boxes because the heat energy generated can actually damage living cells and tissue.

This week experiment with alternative methods to reheat food, such as the stovetop, oven or toaster oven. The extra time it takes will preserve vital nutrients needed to sustain health.

TIP: If you pack your lunch and need to avoid the office microwave oven, consider investing in a good quality thermos.

Make some observations about alternative methods of heating food.

#31

Read Food Labels

What do soy lecithin, modified food starch, dipotassium phosphate and red 40 all have in common? They are all substances found in processed foods. Do you know what they are, why they're in your food and what they can do to your health? Maybe not.

The ability to review packaged food labels is extremely important. Manufactured foods are riddled with chemicals that are detrimental to your health. Chances are, if you cannot pronounce an ingredient or buy it in your supermarket, your body does not recognize it and it is causing harm.

This week research how to read food labels and look up unfamiliar ingredient names. Practice this skill with everything you eat.

How did this experiment make you conscious of what you eat? What did you learn from reading food labels?

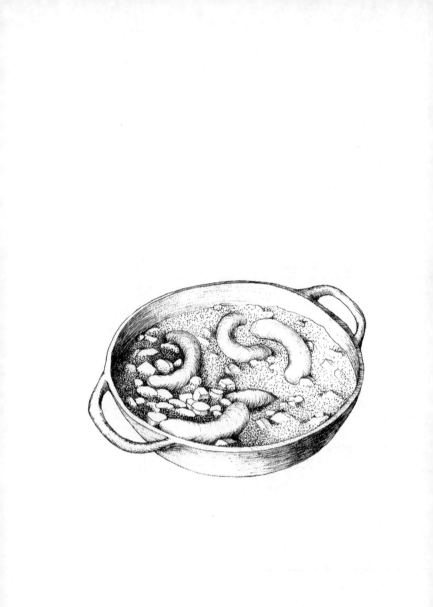

#32

Try a New Recipe

The ability to prepare nourishing food is essential to good health. It's been said that if you can read, you can cook; however, it doesn't always feel that simple. Experiencing joy in the kitchen takes practice. One way to keep the creative juices flowing is to regularly bring new recipes into the fold.

There is no shortage of amazing recipes, so play some inspiring music, pour a glass of wine (if you're so inclined), take a deep breath and try at least two new recipes this week.

Write a few sentences about your experiences.

#33

Visualize

Your mind is a powerful tool. For 5-10 minutes each morning or evening, sit in a relaxed position, close your eyes, maybe play some soothing music, take a few deep breaths and visualize only the day ahead.

Visualize the day in detail from waking up to going to bed. Imagine the day's events being successful and rewarding. Envision yourself smiling and feeling full of love, confidence, joy and courage.

Notice how this simple experiment alters your day.

#34

Smile Like the Mona Lisa

While there is controversy around the meaning of the Mona Lisa's enigmatic smile, there is something to be said about the subtle lure of it. We're attracted to some people for obvious reasons and drawn to others for more elusive reasons. The latter group possesses a certain "je ne sais quoi," but it is most likely their "good energy" to which you're attracted.

This week, experiment with enhancing your energetic attraction by dawning a Mona Lisa smile. Notice if people smile at you more, talk to you more, or compliment you more. And how does your subtle smile affect your own mood? Studies have shown that you can enhance your mental and emotional state by simply smiling.

What did you experience with this experiment?

#35

Think about it

Ponder the following question and journal about your conclusions:

Is your goal in life to be happy or to avoid unhappiness?

#36

Eat Free of Distractions

When you engage in distracted eating, it is easy to tune out, overeat and miss the entire experience. It's like driving somewhere and not recalling the drive. When you eat free of distraction, you truly taste, smell and feel your food. This helps you tap into hunger signals.

This week focus on your food and eat free of distractions in a calm environment. Avoid stressful conversations, put down your smart phone, close your book, turn off the TV and shut down your laptop.

Note your experiences.

#37

Practice Letting Go

Do you need to let go of a person, a habit or thought that no longer serves you?

What prevents you from letting go and moving forward? What would happen if you stopped resisting and simply allowed things to be just as they are? Would you lose a sense of control or be forced to face the truth? And what do you gain by not letting go? Do you hold on to resentment, for example, as a way to protect yourself?

This week, notice what you are holding on to, determine how or why it serves you or doesn't serve you and practice letting it go. You might be asking, "How do I let something go?" Practice an imagery exercise to sever those ties. For example, imagine letting go of someone or something like you would release a balloon into the sky. Or imagine holding a large pair of scissors and cutting the imaginary strings that tie you negatively to something or someone.

Spend some time documenting your experiences with letting go.

#38

Practice Pre-Meal Gratitude

From the farmers to the grocery store clerk, many people work to bring food to your plate. An animal may have even given its life to provide you nourishment.

Take a moment before every meal this week to recognize and thank the people and the animal that made your meal possible.

Be grateful for the life-giving nutrients contained in your food. You are fortunate to have this meal.

How does expressing pre-meal gratitude change your dining experience?

#39

Liberate Your Lymph

You probably know that our body's lymph nodes are important for health; however, you may not know that they are filtration points in a vast network called the lymphatic system. Inside this network, lymph fluid, containing infection-fighting white blood cells, circulates 24/7. It rids your body of toxins, microorganisms and other invaders.

In modern life, this cleansing process is a big job because much of today's food and drink contain toxins. Air quality is also more toxic than ever. When the burden becomes too great for your lymphatic system, the entire system becomes sluggish and clogged.

In addition to eating high quality foods, maintaining a consistent exercise program and managing stress levels, you can assist your lymphatic system with dry skin brushing.

Unlike the heart, the lymph system has no pump, therefore; it needs to be stimulated in order to circulate. Dry skin brushing is an effective and invigorating technique to stimulate lymph movement. Dry skin brushes are sold at most health food stores or easily found online.

Here are a few dry skin brushing tips to get you started:

- Buy a brush made from natural fibers; not plastic.
- Use only on dry skin; never wet.
- Brush arms, legs, abdominals and buttocks.
- Brush towards the heart; never away.
- Brush vigorously and with as much pressure as you can tolerate.

Pamper your lymph system this week by experimenting with daily dry skin brushing.

Document your experience here.

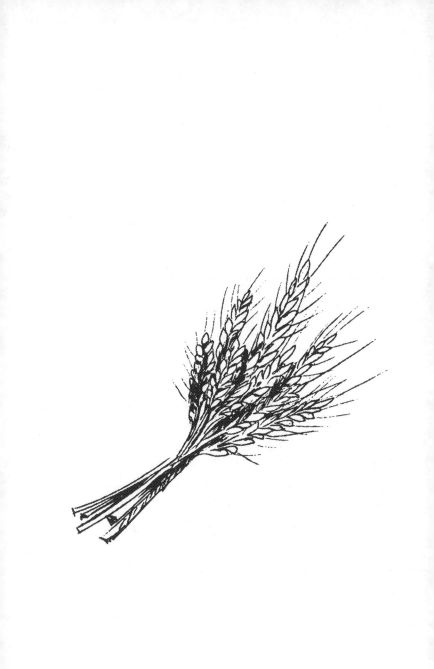

#40

Go Grain Free

Grains come in many forms and are common staples in many people's diets. Grains fall into one of two categories, refined or unrefined.

Refined grains have been stripped of nutrients and fiber, leaving only starch and a small amount of protein. These grains include white rice, white bread, white pasta, all foods made with white flour and processed foods like breakfast cereals, tortillas, baked goods and many sweets. These grains have no place in a healthy diet and should not be consumed.

Unrefined grains are a better choice. Although they are nutrient- and fiber-rich, these may still cause blood sugar issues and weight gain if eaten in excess. Unrefined grains include whole wheat, brown rice, rye, amaranth, barley, buckwheat, oats, quinoa and wild rice.

All grains contain anti-nutrients that interfere with digestion and render them unavailable to the body. Many people find that a grain-free diet improves digestion, gas and bloating and promotes weight loss.

For this week, experiment with eating grain-free and notice how you feel.

#41

Have a Dance Party!

Liberate your soul by dancing with abandon in the privacy of your own space. Pick the time, place and music and just move to the rhythm in your own unique way. No judgment, no conformity, no rules, just whatever feels right.

This exercise allows you to express yourself and provides creative space and awakening. Experiment with dancing every day this week.

How did your dance parties make you feel?

#42

Journal It

Choose one of the following thoughts and journal about it. If you enjoy writing, choose a different one each day!

1. Happy place.
2. It is what it is.
3. Choose joy.
4. Perseverance.
5. Love is all around you.

#43

Cut Out Caffeine

There are benefits to eliminating or reducing caffeine consumption.

You may realize you're more reliant on caffeine than you think. This week challenge yourself to either decrease or cut out caffeine. Notice if this change affects your mood, energy levels, hydration and sleep patterns.

There are several ways to perform this experiment. Either go cold turkey or reduce consumption a little more each day. You can swap caffeinated beverages for lower or no caffeine alternatives like lemon water, kombucha, freshly pressed juices, green teas and herbal teas.

Note: you may experience withdrawal symptoms such as headache or fatigue—these are normal detox symptoms and should pass as your body adjusts. Hang in there.

What did you learn about yourself this week?

#44

Neti Pot

Regular nasal irrigation with a neti pot naturally cleanses and protects the nasal passages—one of your immune system's first lines of defense. Rinsing debris and mucus away reduces seasonal allergies, runny nose and sinus congestion.

If you don't already own one, neti pots can be found in health food stores and pharmacies or purchased online. This week, use a neti pot daily.

Did you notice any changes?

#45

Maintain Your Friendships

Our friendships shape who we become. When we are young, friendships teach us to share and work together. As we age, friendships open us to new hobbies, worldviews and interests. They also serve as sounding boards for advice and perspective.

Friendships enhance our lives by teaching us about ourselves and the world. They serve as a link to our past, give us a sense of purpose, and are sources of joy and entertainment.

Like a beautiful garden, friendships need attention to flourish.

This week, make an effort to connect with an old friend. Pick up the phone or meet in-person. You could even write a letter or book a flight to visit someone you haven't seen in years.

What did you do?

#46

Remove Artificial and Refined Sugar

Unless it comes without an ingredient label, most foods contain added sugars or artificial sweeteners. In the early 1800s, Americans consumed 10 pounds of sugar per person per year. Today, the average American consumes 180 pounds per person per year. It's no wonder that lifestyle diseases like obesity, diabetes, heart disease and cancer are increasing.

For this week avoid all refined sugars and artificial sweeteners. These ingredients confuse your brain into never feeling full, contribute to weight gain, negatively impact your mood and cause blood sugar highs and lows.

Read all food labels and know the many names of refined sugar and artificial sweeteners such as barley malt, beet sugar, brown sugar, cane sugar/juice, corn syrup, date sugar, dextrose, disaccharides, fructose, fruit juice concentrate, glucose syrup, glycerol, high fructose corn syrup (HFCS), lactose, maltodextrin, maltose, mannitol, molasses, polydextrose, rice extract, saccharin, sorbitol, sucrose, xylitol, acesulfame-K, alitame, aspartame, cyclamates, neohesperdine, neotame, rebiana, saccharin, sucralose, and thaumatin.

You might be surprised at how many hidden refined and artificial sugars are in food.

What did you learn from this experiment?

#47

Get Grateful

Your life is filled with abundance, even if you're too busy or stressed to realize. Practicing gratitude shifts mental focus to the good things in life—no matter how big or small. Gratitude lends itself to positive thinking and puts you in a position to accept even more abundance. *And who wouldn't want more!?*

At bedtime for the next week, write down three positive things that happened during the day. Notice how your mindset shifts the more you practice gratitude.

#48

Curb Your Carbs

Carbohydrates are the most diverse (and confusing) group of macronutrients. At a basic level, carbohydrates contain sugars, starches and fibers used by the body for quick energy.

There are two main groups of carbohydrates, simple and complex.

Simple carbohydrates are broken down quickly and contain little fiber, vitamins and minerals. These include most baked goods, white rice, white bread, some dairy products and sugary foods like sodas and candy.

Complex carbohydrates contain fiber, vitamins and minerals, take longer to digest and are healthier for you. Examples include fruits, vegetables, brown rice, whole grain breads, oatmeal and legumes. Complex carbohydrates are an important part of a daily diet; however, some people are unable to digest many of the processed complex carbohydrates like breads, grains and legumes. When they eat these foods, it results in digestive distress like gas, bloating and pain.

For this week, experiment with eating ONLY fruit and vegetable carbohydrates. Make sure to eat plenty of proteins and good fats, but avoid all breads, grains, pastas, beans, legumes, processed foods and sugary sweets. Your meals and snacks should be comprised of proteins, fats, fruits and vegetables only.

Notice how a week with fewer carbohydrates makes you feel.

#49

Pamper Yourself

In order to care for others, you must first care for yourself. Has it been a while since you've done something nice for yourself? When is the last time you put your needs ahead of someone else's? It's your week to put yourself first and indulge.

Carve out time to pamper yourself this week with a manicure, pedicure, bubble bath, massage, nap, workout or whatever makes you feel special. You deserve it.

How did it feel?

#50

Compliment Others

Compliments are meant to be shared, yet we often withhold them. Why is that?

In every interaction this week, find an authentic way to make the other person feel good. Maybe he's wearing a great outfit. Maybe you like her earrings. Maybe their child is waiting respectfully while you visit. Maybe the person just has a glow.

Find something amazing about the person and let him/ her know.

Document your experience.

#51

Oil Pull

Oil pulling is an ancient Indian practice. Swishing a tablespoon of oil in your mouth for 10-20 minutes gives you fresher breath, fewer cavities and a whiter smile.

Coconut oil is naturally anti-microbial, making it a great oral detoxifier. Once a day, place one tablespoon of coconut oil in your mouth, allow it to liquefy and swish it around the gums and through the teeth. Work up to 20 minutes of daily oil pulling for maximum benefits.

Don't forget: when finished, discard the oil properly. Spit it into an old shampoo bottle or into the trash but never down the drain.

How'd it go?

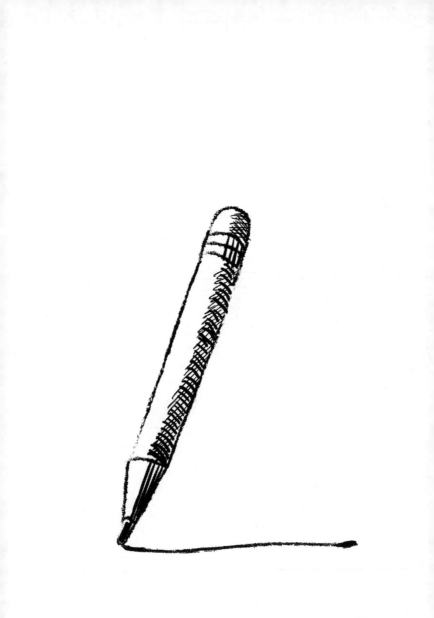

#52

Write Your Eulogy

What will your eulogy say? How will you be remembered?

Spend time this week crafting a memorial to your former self. How would you describe, commemorate and celebrate you?

Endnotes

1   *Merriam-Webster's Desk Dictionary.* (1995). Versailles, Kentucky: Merriam-Webster, Inc.

2   *New Oxford American Dictionary* (3rd ed.). (2010). Oxford, New York: Oxford University Press, Inc.

About the Authors

Lily Milkovic and Jenny Swain are close friends and Certified Nutritional Therapy Practitioners living in Texas. Both share a passion for helping others find optimal health. In their spare time, Lily enjoys time with friends, yoga and travel while Jenny loves to read, cook and spend time with her kids.

Printed in the United States
By Bookmasters